Published By Robert Corbin

@ Alfred Lowry

Wheat Belly Diet: Easy And Wheat -Free Recipes

To health and weight-loss Plan

All Right RESERVED

ISBN 978-1-990666-91-9

I0554706

TABLE OF CONTENTS

Sour Cherry Pancakes

Ingredients:

- ¼ cup quick-cooking oats

- 2 tsp baking soda

- 1 tsp salt

- 2 eggs, beaten

- 2 cups buttermilk

- ½ cup almonds, halved

- ½ cup Greek yogurt

- ½ cup dried sweetened sour cherries

- 1 cinnamon stick

- ½ cup maple syrup

- 1 ½ cups all-purpose flour

- ¼ cup whole-wheat flour

Directions:

1. Add the cherries, water & cinnamon stick to a saucepan.

2. Bring this mixture to the boil over a high heat. Lower the temperature and leave to simmer for 6-8 minutes.

3. Gradually add the syrup, then remove the saucepan from the heat and set aside for later.

4. Combine the oats, flours, eggs & buttermilk in a mixing bowl.

5. Pour in the saucepan contents and beat everything together until a moist batter is produced.

6. Using low-calorie cooking spray, grease a large non-stick iron skillet.

7. Heat the skillet over a high heat for 2-3 minutes.

Grilled Peaches With Coconut Cream

Ingredients:

- 1 teaspoon vanilla

- 1 can coconut milk, refrigerated

- 1/4 cup chopped walnuts

- 3 medium ripe peaches, cut in half with pit removed

- Cinnamon to taste

Directions:

1. Place Peaches On The Grill With The Cut Side Down First.
2. Grill On Medium-Low Heat Until Soft, About 3-5 Minutes On Each Side.
3. Scoop Cream Off The Top Of The Can Of Chilled Coconut Milk.
4. Whip Together Coconut Cream And Vanilla With Handheld Mixer.

5. Drizzle Over Each Peach. Top With Cinnamon And Chopped Walnuts To Garnish.

No-Bake Mini Pumpkin Bites

Ingredients:

For Crust:

- 1 tablespoon coconut oil

- 1 tablespoon REAL maple syrup or raw h2y

- 2 pinches of Celtic sea salt

- 1 cup hazelnuts

- 1/2 cup raw pumpkin seeds

- 8 date, pitted

For Filling:

- 1/4 teaspoon cinnamon powder

- 1/4 teaspoon ginger powder

- 1/8 teaspoon allspice

5

- 1/8 teaspoon clove powder

- 1 cup cooked pumpkin puree

- 1/2 cup coconut butter

- 2 tablespoon coconut oil

- 3 tablespoon REAL maple syrup or raw h2y

- 1/2 teaspoon vanilla extract

For Chocolate Drizzle:

- 2 tablespoons coconut oil

- 2 tablespoons raw cacao

- 3 tablespoons REAL maple syrup or raw h2y

- 2 tablespoons coconut butter

- Pinch or 2 of salt

Directions:

1. To make the crust: Line mini muffin tins with unbleached mini paper liners .

2. Process all crust Ingredients: in a food processor until well combined and resembles a coarse flour.

3. Spoon 1 and 1/2 teaspoon of mixture into each of the 24 mini cups.

4. Use your thumb to press down mixture firmly to create a solid bottom layer for these cute little yummies.

5. Place in freezer to harden.

6. To make filling: Melt coconut butter and coconut oil in a double boiler.

7. Remove from heat and add rest of filling Ingredients:.

8. Go ahead and mix it up real good here until creamy smooth.

9. Remove crusts from freezer and spoon about 3/4 TBS of filling over your prepared crusts.

10. Return to freezer to harden, at least 2 hours.

11. To make chocolate drizzle: Once mini bites have hardened, gently melt coconut butter and coconut oil in a double boiler.

12. Remove from heat and add rest of drizzle Ingredients:.

13. Allow to cool slightly to thicken. Pour into small plastic bag, cut a TINY hole in the corner, and drizzle over treats in any fashion that you want.

14. Now it's time to enjoy these amazing delights. Store leftovers in freezer as they are best cold.

Chocolate Hazelnut Cups

Ingredients:

- 2 10 ounce bag of dark chocolate chips

- 3 tablespoons of coconut oil--2 for the chocolate and 2 for the nuts

- 3 10 ounce bags of chopped hazelnuts or almonds, or any nut

Directions:

1. Melt the chocolate over low heat, stirring in a tablespoon of coconut oil once the chips are melted.

2. While your chocolate is melting, add the hazelnuts to a food processor and blend.

3. That's seriously it. It takes a few minutes, but you'll have hazelnut butter before you know it.

4. Throw in a tablespoon of coconut oil for good measure.
5. Spoon some melted chocolate into the bottoms of your candy molds.
6. Add a bit of hazelnut butter. Top it with another spoonful of chocolate. Stick them in the freezer until they've hardened and pop them out.
7. Store them in the refrigerator. Share them with some2 you really like.

Coconut Chocolate Tart

Ingredients:

- Sweetener – should be equivalent to 2 cup of sugar

- 8 oz 100% chocolate

- 14 oz heavy cream or canned coconut milk

- 3 separated eggs

- 1/2 teaspoon vanilla extract

- 2 1/2 cups shredded coconut, unsweetened

- 2 teaspoons divided ground cinnamon

- 1/4 cup almond flour/meal

- 1/4 cup melted butter or coconut oil

Directions:

1. While preheating the oven to 350F, grease a 9-inch pie pan.
2. In a medium-sized bowl, combine your almond flour/meal, coconut, butter/oil, 1/4 cup sweetener and 1/2 tsp cinnamon and mix them thoroughly.
3. Transfer the mixture to your greased pie pan.
4. Spread it evenly on the bottom of the pie pan, and partially up the sides.
5. Bake this for 10 minutes, until the edges are lightly browned. Remove from the oven and allow to cool.
6. While your coconut shell is baking, heat your chocolate and cream or coconut milk over medium heat in a saucepan, until the chocolate melts. Stir in your remaining sweetener.

7. Take care not to overheat the mixture. Remove it from heat.

8. Whip three egg whites until they form stiff peaks.

9. Reduce your speed and blend in the egg yolks, remaining cinnamon and vanilla.

10. Add your chocolate mixture with a spoon and blend it in with this mix gradually.

11. Pour your chocolate mixture into the coconut shell, and then bake for 15 additional minutes.

12. Remove from oven and allow to cool.

13. Refrigerate until it sets. It is then ready to serve and enjoy.

Nutty Crunch Raisin Bars

Ingredients:

- 1/2 cup pumpkin seeds, raw

- 1 teaspoon vanilla extract

- 1 cup whey protein

- 1/2 cup almond butter, at room temperature

- 1/2 cup raisins, dried

- Sweetener that is equivalent to 1/2 cup of sugar

- 1/2 cup water

- 2 cups unsweetened coconut, shredded

- 2 teaspoons cinnamon, ground

- 1/4 cup melted coconut oil

- 1/2 cup walnut fragments

- 1/4 teaspoon sea salt

Directions:

1. Preheat your oven to 300F.

2. Combine cinnamon and coconut, and mix in a large bowl.

3. Mix vanilla and melted coconut oil in a smaller bowl. Add this to your coconut mixture.

4. Mix this thoroughly and coat the coconut with oil.

5. Spread the mixture in a thin layer on a baking sheet.

6. Bake for five minutes, then remove and toss lightly with a spoon.

7. Continue to heat for an addition 3 or three minutes, until the mixture has browned lightly, and immediately remove.

8. The idea is to remove the mixture as soon as it starts browning, or the coconut will burn.

9. Transfer the toasted coconut to the large bowl.

10. Mix in pumpkin seeds, almond butter, water, salt, sweetener, whey protein, raisins and walnuts and combine.

11. Shape this mixture into bars and place on wax paper or parchment paper.

12. Store them in the refrigerator.

13. Giving up wheat doesn't mean giving up tasty meals and snacks, especially since you won't be counting calories – just preparing foods without wheat.

14. Add ¼ cup pancake batter to the skillet. Sprinkle the batter with a pinch of almonds and cook for 2-3 minutes per side.

15. Repeat this process for all the batter, then serve.

Wheat & Gluten Free Blueberry Muffins Recipe

Ingredients:

- 1/2 tsp grated organic lemon peel
  non-organic lemons have waxed
  skins

- 1 dessert apple, peeled, chopped
  and cooked with 1 tbsp water, then
  mashed to a purée or use 125ml
  [1/2 cup] unsweetened readymade
  apple purée

- 1 large egg, beaten

- 4 tsp light olive oil or flavourless oil

- 100ml milk substitute: almond,
  rice, soy milks

- 1/4 tsp vanilla extract

- 125g fresh blueberries not frozen

- 6 large paper muffin cases

- 70g brown rice flour

- 45g tapioca flour

- 45g potato flour

- 1 1⁄4 tsp baking powder

- 1⁄2 tsp xanthan gum

- 1⁄2 tsp unflavoured vegetarian gelatine we used Agar flakes

- 30g sugar

Directions:

1. Preheat oven: 200°C, 400°F, Gas 6
2. Mix together the rice, tapioca and potato flours, baking powder, xanthan gum, vegetarian gelatine, sugar, salt and lemon peel.

3. Mix the apple puree with the egg, oil, milk and vanilla. Mix this into the dry ingredients so that you get a lumpy batter.
4. Gently fold the blueberries into the mixture, then divide equally into the 6 muffin cases in a muffin tray.
5. Bake for 25 minutes, check they are cooked by sticking a toothpick in the centre, if it comes out clean they are done.
6. Leave to cool on a baking tray.
7. These muffins are delicious either hot or cold, and will keep in an airtight container for a couple of days.
8. They also freeze well, line an airtight freezer container with waxed paper or baking parchment, place muffins inside and cover with some more waxed or parchment paper.
9. Use frozen blueberry muffins within a month.

Wheat & Gluten Free Carrot Cake

Ingredients:

- 115g fresh dates, finely chopped

- 150g carrot, grated

- 175g pear, peeled, cored and pureed

- 175g gluten free flour

- 2 tsp baking powder

- 2 tsp ground cinnamon

- 1 tsp grated nutmeg

- 115g low fat spread, butter or margarine

- 3 large eggs, beaten

- 1/2 tsp mixed spice

- 1/4 tsp salt

Directions:

1. Preheat oven: 190°C, 375°F, Gas 5
2. Line a 16-18cm 6-7" spring form cake tin with baking parchment.
3. Cream the low fat spread, butter or margarine in a large mixing bowl, gradually beat in the eggs, the mixture may curdle at this stage, but this will not spoil the cake.
4. Mix in the dates, carrot and pear, mix well.
5. Sift the gluten free flour, baking powder, spices and salt, then gently fold into the fruit mixture, making sure it is thoroughly mixed without losing the beaten in air.
6. Spoon the mixture into the cake tin and bake for 55-60 minutes.
7. To check if cooked insert a clean toothpick into the middle of the cake, it should come out clean.

8. Remove cake from tin and allow to cool on a wire rack.

9. Serve with whipped cream, ice cream or Greek yogurt as a refreshing dessert after dinner, or as a cake for afternoon tea.

10. This cake keeps well in an airtight container for 2-3 days.

Cauliflower Soup

Ingredients:

- ½ a teaspoon of coriander

- 2 tablespoons of Harissa paste

- 1l of vegetable stock

- 50g toasted flaked almonds

- 1 large cauliflower

- 2 tablespoons of olive oil

- ½ a teaspoon of cinnamon

- ½ a teaspoon of cumin

Directions:

1. Chop the cauliflower into florets. In a frying pan, warm 3 tablespoons of olive oil for 2-3 minutes.

2. Next add cinnamon, cumin, coriander and Harissa paste and fry for 2 more minutes.
3. Afterwards, add the cauliflower florets, vegetable stock and flaked almonds.
4. Cover and leave to cook for 20 minutes. Blend with a hand processor and serve.

Mediterranean Salsa

Ingredients:

- 140g black beans

- Lime juice

- ½ bunch of coriander

- 2 tablespoons of olive oil

- 250g sweet corn

- Spring Onions

Directions:

1. Slice spring onions and chop the coriander bunch, including the stalks.
2. Bring a saucepan of water to the boil, add the black beans and leave to simmer for 45 minutes.

3. Remove the black beans and combine them with the sweet corn, spring onions, and coriander.

4. Drizzle with a little olive oil and lime juice.

Harvest Pumpkin Custard

Ingredients:

Pumpkin Mix:

- 3/4 cup raw h2y

- 1 teaspoon pumpkin pie spice

- 1/4 teaspoon salt

- 1 can pumpkin puree

- 1 cup coconut cream

Coconut Whipped Cream:

- 1 can coconut milk, full fat

- 1/4 teaspoon vanilla optional

- 1/4 teaspoon cinnamon optional

Crumble Mixture:

- 3/4 cup hazelnut flour

- 2 teaspoon cinnamon

- 2 tablespoon coconut sugar

Directions:

Pumpkin Mix:

1. In a large metal bowl, combine the pumpkin puree, coconut cream, raw h2y, pumpkin pie spice, and salt. Mix until thoroughly combined.

Coconut Whipped Cream:

2. To make the coconut whipped cream: do not open the can of coconut milk.

3. Place in the refrigerator for at least 2 hours ideally overnight.

4. Open the can of coconut milk and scoop out thickened coconut cream on top into a bowl. If preferred, you can drink the coconut water or save it for a smoothie.

5. Optional: add cinnamon and vanilla.

6. Finally, whip the coconut cream with a whisk or electric beater until it begins to thicken.

Crumble Mixture:

7. In another small bowl, combine the hazelnut flour, the cinnamon, and the coconut sugar. Mixed until combined.
8. In a tall class, mason jars or a large glass dish, alternate the layers of pumpkin mix, coconut cream, and the crumble mixture, ending with the crumble mixture on top. You can choose to in 2 round of layers or multiple layers.

Chico-Coconut Drops

Ingredients:

- 2 tablespoon raw h2y

- 1/4 cup almond butter

- 1 cup coconut flakes, unsweetened

- 3 tablespoon coconut oil

- 1/2 cup dark chocolate chips

- 1/4 cup unsweetened cocoa powder

Directions:

1. In a microwave safe bowl, add the coconut oil and chocolate chips. In small increments of time so that the chocolate doesn't burn, cook the mixture at 30 second intervals until the chis are melted.

2. Make sure to stir between each of the 30 second intervals.

3. You can even turn down you power level to further ensure no burning.

4. Once mixture is melted, stir in the cocoa powder, h2y, and almond butter. Mix until smooth.

5. Then add the coconut and stir until coated.

6. Drop the batter in scoops on a parchment paper lined baking sheet.

7. Refrigerate the cookies until they are firm. Store leftover in the fridge.

Sweet Peach Crisp

Ingredients:

- 2 tbsp. Butter

- 1 ¼ c. almond flour, whitened

- Salt

- 1 kg. peaches, cut

- 1 tbsp. maple syrup

- ½ tsp. vanilla concentrate

Directions:

1. Lay out the cut peaches into a heating dish.
2. Blend the almond flour and salt in a sustenance processor.
3. At that point, beat with the butter, maple syrup, and vanilla. Pour mixture over the peaches.

4. Prepare in the oven for roughly 45 minutes at 350 degrees.

5. Give it a chance to cool before serving.

Sweet Macaroons

Ingredients:

- ¼ cup nectar

- 2 tbsp. Additional virgin coconut oil

- 1 tbsp. Vanilla concentrate

- 1 ½ cup destroyed coconut, unsweetened

- 1 tbsp. Coconut flour

- Salt

Directions:

1. Blend the destroyed coconuts with the coconut flour in the nourishment processor. Join with nectar, coconut oil, salt, and vanilla concentrate by beating.

2. Shape mixture into a ball. Spot balls into a preparing sheet for heating.

3. For a most extreme of 7 minutes, bake at 350 degrees.

4. Let the macaroons cool for 3 or three hours prior to serving.

Wheat-Free Garlic Bread

Ingredients:

Wet:

- 2 ½ cups of warm water around 105-110°F

- 1 teaspoon h2y

- 2 tablespoons maple syrup

- 2 ¼ teaspoons of dynamic dry yeast

- 2 tablespoons of additional

- 1/3 cup of entire psyllium husks

- 1/3 cup of ground chia seeds

- olive oil in addition to extra for topping

Dry:

- 1 cup sorghum flour

- ½ cup sweet rice flour

- 1 cup teff flour

- ½ cup almond meal

- 1 ½ teaspoons of ocean salt

Directions:

1. Preheat the stove to 400° Fahrenheit.

2. Put the warm water in a bowl. Consolidate a teaspoon of h2y and the yeast and whisk them together.

3. Leave the blend for around 5-10 minutes to allow the yeast to actuate.

4. The combination ought to turn out to be effervescent or frothy. In the event that this doesn't occur, dispose of the combination and start over.

5. While the yeast is being actuated, you can begin blending the dry fixings in a major bowl.

6. When the yeast is enacted, include the maple syrup, olive oil, psyllium husks, and ground chia seeds into the blend.

7.   Leave the blend for around 2-3 minutes this is significant, so watch an opportunity to let the psyllium and the chia seeds discharge a gelatin-like substance. Whisk these together.

8. Pour every 2 of the wet fixings into the bowl with the dry fixings.

9. Combine everything as 2 utilizing a wooden spoon until the combination turns out to be thick.

10. On a floured wooden board, manipulate the batter to blend in the flour.

11. Add the newly slashed garlic as you work. Add a greater amount of the sorghum and teff flours, a little at a time.

12. Keep adding until the mixture keeps yet is still a piece tacky to the touch.

13. Make a ball with the batter and set it back into the enormous bowl.

14. Cover it with a clammy towel. Place the bowl in a warm spot with the goal that the batter rises.

15. Some put the bowl on a pot that has warm water.

16. Allow it to ascend until the batter is multiplied in size.

17. When the mixture has risen, put a pizza st2 inside the broiler.

18. Set a container of water on the base rack, just underneath the pizza st2. You can utilize a 8x8-inch glass container loaded up with water about ¾ of the way.

19. Punch the mixture down and spread it out onto a wooden board that has been gently floured.

20. Ply it for about a moment and afterward structure it into a ball. Put the mixture on a square piece of material paper.

21. Utilizing a sharp blade, make a shallow example on top a spasm tac-toe design. Shower the top with olive oil,

22. and afterward sprinkle with sesame and poppy seeds. Allow the mixture to ascend for 30 minutes more in a warm place.

23. Carefully lift the material paper with the batter, and put it on the st2 inside the stove. Prepare the bread for 40 minutes.
    Remove the bread from the stove once cooked, and let it cool for around 30-an hour prior to cutting it.

24. The bread is still a piece sticky in surface when hot and recently out of the oven.

Dried Fruit Sc2s

Ingredients:

- ½ teaspoon of xanthan gum

- 2 teaspoons of baking powder

- ¼ teaspoon nutmeg this is optional

- ½ teaspoon of salt

- ¾ cup of diced dried organic product relies upon your inclination 2 enormous eggs

- ½ cup spread, cold

- 2 ¼ cups of earthy colored rice flour

- ¼ cup of sugar

- 1/3 cup milk, cold

- 1 teaspoon of vanilla concentrate wheat and gluten-free

Directions:

1. Preheat your broiler to 400 degrees Fahrenheit.
2. Oil a baking sheet or line it with material paper.
3. You can likewise utilize a partiti2d sc2 prospect, yet you need to lube it appropriately in front of time.
4. Whisk the flour, thickener, sugar, salt, baking powder, and nutmeg together.
5. Ensure that everything is blended well. Add in the virus spread until the subsequent combination is brittle for all intents and purposes and texture.
6. Add in the dry blend into the brittle mixture. In another bowl, include the vanilla, milk, and the eggs.
7. Blend until frothy.

8. Add in the past combination into the dry combination.
9. Mix everything great. Everything ought to be very much mixed.
10. The subsequent mixture ought to be exceptionally tacky and cohesive.
11. Drop the batter onto the sc2 skillet or baking sheet, around 1/3 of a cup at a time.
12. In the event that you decide not to have dried organic product, decrease how much mixture you add onto the sc2 skillet or baking sheet, pretty much ¼ of a cup in particular.
13. Pass on the mixture to rest for around 15 minutes.
14. Add cinnamon sugar or shimmering sugar on the sc2s prior to baking them, on the off chance that you like.
15. Heat them for 15-20 minutes, or until the sc2s are brilliant brown in shading.

16. Take them out from the stove and let them cool for 5 minutes.

17. You can add spread and jam for an ideal treat!

Roasted Chicken

Ingredients:

- 2 teaspoons onion powder

- 1/3 cup margarine, divided

- 5/8 stalk celery

- 3 pound whole chicken, giblets removed

- Salt and black pepper to taste

Directions:

1. Preheat oven to 350o F.
2. Place chicken in a roasting pan and season generously inside and out with salt and pepper and onion powder.
3. Place 3 tablespoons margarine in the cavity of the chicken.
4. Arrange remaining margarine on outer side.

5. Cut celery into pieces and place in the cavity of the chicken.
6. Bake for 2 hour and 15 minutes in oven to a internal temperature of 180 degrees F.
7. Remove from heat and sprinkle with margarine and lard.
8. Cover with foil and let stand 30 minutes before serving.

Orange Salmon

Ingredients:

- Salt to taste

- 1 salmon filets

- olive oil

- 1 tbsp.

  fresh orange juice

- ½ tbsp. h2y

- ½ tbsp. fresh cilantro

Directions:

1. Mix orange juice and h2y in a cup. Place the cup in the microwave and heat for 15-20 seconds.
2. Cut the salmon fillet into small chunks.
3. Preheat oven to 450o F. Place a large nonstick skillet in the oven for about 10 minutes.

4. Remove and sprinkle the pan with a little olive oil. Place fillets in the pan.
5. Pour the sauce over the fillets and wrap the pan in the oven.
6. Bake for about 3 minutes.
7. Toss and cook both sides sprinkling sauce often over the fish.
8. Once cooked, remove from oven and sprinkle with cilantro.

Dark Choco Popsicles

Ingredients:

- 1 tbsp. maple syrup

- 2 cups coconut milk

- 2 scoops protein powder

- 1/3 cup unsweetened dark cocoa powder

- 1 tsp. vanilla extract

Directions:

1. Combine the coconut milk and chocolate into a sauce pan and then heat over low-mmedium fire for a few minutes.
2. Transfer the chocolate mixture into a blender and then add the remaining recipes.
3. Pour the mixture into popsicle molds or ice trays and freeze.

No-Bake Blueberry Cheesecake

Ingredients:

- 2½ tsp. gelatin

- 1 cup stevia

- 6 oz. fresh blueberries

- 1½ cups water

- 1 cup ica

- 8 oz. sour cream

- 8 oz. cream cheese

- ½ cup stevia

- 1 tsp. vanilla extract

Crust Recipe

- 1 tsp. powdered cinnamon

- ½tsp. salt

- 1 egg

- 1½cup almond meal

- 4 oz. organic butter melted

Directions:

1. In a mixing bowl, combine the almond meal, salt, and cinnamon. Combine thoroughly and then add the egg and melted butter.

2. Take a 9"pie plate and spread the crust on the pie mold using a large spoon.

3. Whip the cream cheese, sour cream, vanilla and stevia using a handheld electronic mixer. Blend for 3 mins. or until creamy.

4. Pour the cheese mixture into the pie crust and freeze for a minimum for 30 mins.

5. In a sauce pan over low fire, place water and gelatin and stir for 5 minutes. Add the stevia and heat for several minutes until al the gelatin are dissolved.

6. Add the blueberries and then remove from heat. Add the ice and stir.
7. Let it cool for 30 mins.
8. Pour the gelatin mixture into the pie and then refrigerate for minimum of 2 hours or overnight.

Avocado-Turkey Wraps

Ingredients:

- ¼ cup of bean sprouts

- ½ of Hass avocado sliced thinly

- Leaves of baby spinach or lettuce shredded

- Flaxseed wrap recipe will follow

- 3-4 slices of deli roast turkey

- 2 slices of Swiss cheese

- 1 tablespoon of mayonnaise you can also use wasabi mayonnaise, mustard or no-sugar salad dressing

Directions:

1. Place swiss cheese and turkey on the center of your wrap. Add layers of avocado, spinach and bean sprouts.

2. Top it with a dollop or scoop of mayonnaise.

3. Roll the wrap. Serve and enjoy!

To Make The Flaxseed Wrap

Ingredients:

- ¼ teaspoon of onion powder

- 1 tablespoon of coconut oil add more to grease the pans; melted

- 1 tablespoon of water

- 1 large sized egg

- 3 tablespoons of flaxseeds ground

- ¼ teaspoon of baking powder

- A pinch of sea salt you can also use celery salt

Directions:

1. Using a small sized bowl, combine baking powder, flaxseeds, paprika, onion powder and salt.

2. Add a tablespoon of coconut oil and stir a little.
3. Add the egg and a tablespoon of coconut oil.
4. Mix well until it turned to a batter.
5. Using a microwave safe bowl or a pie pan, grease it with the coconut oil.
6. Pour the batter and spread it evenly on the bottom.
7. Cook inside the microwave oven for about 2-3 minutes on high heat until it is cooked. Let cool for about 5 minutes.
8. To remove the wrap, lift using the edge of your spatula. In case it sticks, try to using pancake turner so that it would lose gently on the pan.
9. Flip and place on a plate. Top with your desired filling. Serve and enjoy! This recipe is good for 1 serving only.

No Grain Sushi

Ingredients:

- Sweetener which is equal to 3 teaspoons of sugar

- 2 teaspoons of apple cider vinegar

- ¼ teaspoon of rock salt pink or sea salt gray

- 1 tablespoon of pesto

- 1 tablespoon of yellow mustard prepared

- 3 oz of canned mackerel or herring you can also use a cup of black beans that are cooked, rinsed and drained

- 2 cups of cauliflower steamed and florets are cut to small pieces

- 3 pieces of nori sheets

- ½ cup of cucumber sliced thinly

- ½ cup of carrot sliced thinly

Directions:

1. Combine sweetener, cauliflower, salt and vinegar using your food processor.
2. Pulse until mixture becomes rice like. Place in a bowl. Set aside.
3. In a separate bowl, mix mustard, fish and pesto and mash them until it turned to a paste consistency.
4. Using your sushi roller, lay the nori sheet and spread some thin layer of the cauliflower rice on top of the nori.
5. Leave at least 2 inches on the bottom to allow some space for rolling.
6. Spread another layer of the fish mixture on top of the cauliflower rice.

7. Layer with carrots and cucumber at the center of the nori sheet then roll it firmly and seal the end with a dab of water.

8. Using your sharp knife, cut to an inch size coin. Serve and enjoy!

Curried Quinoa Salad

Ingredients:

- Fresh cilantro 3 tablespoons, chopped

- Currants 3 tablespoons

- English cucumber 1/4 cup finely diced peeled

- Fresh mint 2 teaspoons chopped

- Plain low-fat yogurt 1 carton

- Kosher salt 3/4 teaspoon

- Ripe Mango 1 diced peeled

- Celery 1/2 cup diced

- Olive oil 1 teaspoon

- Madras curry powder 2 teaspoons

- 1 garlic clove crushed

- Quinoa 1 cup, uncooked

- Water 2 cups

- Green onions 1/4 cup thinly sliced

Directions:
1. Place a saucepan over a medium-high heat and add some oil.
2. Add the curry powder and garlic, and while stirring, cook for 1 minute.
3. Add the quinoa, along with 2 cups of water and then boil.
4. Reduce the heat, cover with a lid and simmer for 15 minutes.
5. Turn the heat off, add the salt and let it cool.
6. Add the ripe mango, celery, onions, cilantro, and currants, and then toss gently.
7. Mix the cucumber, yogurt and mint in a small bowl to make a simple Raita sauce.

8. Divide the quinoa salad amongst approx. 6 plates, top with the Raita sauce and serve chilled.

Pork And Eggs

Ingredients:

- Sea salt ¼ teaspoon

- Pepper ¼ teaspoon

- Garlic ¼ teaspoon

- Almond meal or flour 2 tablespoons

- Flax flour 2 tablespoons

- Baking soda 1/2 teaspoon

- Eggs 14

- Celery 3 stalks, chopped

- Red onion 1/2 cup, diced

- Ground pork 1 pound

- Mozzarella 4 ounces, grated

- Butter 2 tablespoons

- Cheddar cheese 2 ounces, grated

Directions:

1. Set the oven to 350 degrees F.
2. In a large skillet, saute the celery, onion, and ground pork.
3. After a minute, add pepper, salt, and garlic to the pepper and mix well.
4. In a separate bowl, add almond flour, flax flour, baking soda, 8 eggs, and grated mozzarella. Whisk and mix well.
5. Pour the batter into a baking dish, and place the cooked pork mixture on it.
6. Sprinkle grated cheddar on top and bake for 20 minutes.
7. Remove from the oven. Add the remaining 6 eggs on top of it. The eggs should be whisked together in a bowl first.
8. Bake again until the egg layer on top is cooked. Then serve.

Wheat Free Pizza

Ingredients:

- Extra-virgin olive oil 1/4 cup

- Sausage 1 lb, bulk or loose

- Onion 1 medium-sized, chopped

- Garlic cloves 2 pieces, minced

- Bell pepper 1/2, chopped

- Dried oregano 1 teaspoon

- Parmesan or Romano cheese 2 tablespoons, grated

- Sugar-free pizza sauce OR marinara sauce 2 cups

- Fresh mozzarella 8 ounces, thinly sliced

For Wheat-Belly Pizza Crust:

- 1/3 tsp. Onion powder

- 1/2 tsp. Sea salt

- 2 eggs

- 1/3 cup extra-virgin olive oil

- 1/2 cup water

- 1 cup shredded mozzarella cheese

- 1 cup almond flour

- 1/4 cup chickpea flour

- 1/4 golden flaxseed

Directions:

1. Put the mozzarella into a food blender and blend until it becomes grain sized.

2. Mix the mozzarella, almonds, chickpea flour, flaxseeds, onion powder, garlic powder, and salt in a large bowl.

3. Then stir in the eggs, oil, and water and mix thoroughly.

4. This will form the dough.

5. Put the dough onto a baking tray lined with parchment paper and flatten it out into a circular pizza shape.

6. Bake for 20 minutes at 350 degrees F.

7. While the crust is baking, place a skillet over medium heat and add 2 tablespoons of olive oil.

8. Put in the garlic and onion, cook for a minute, then add the sausage and cook for a further 10 minutes.

9. Then remove from the heat.

10. Once pizza crust has baked after 20 minutes or so spread the pizza sauce evenly on it.

11. Place the mozzarella, the cooked sausage, oregano, bell pepper, and cheese.
12. Drizzle 2 tablespoons of olive oil on top.
13. Put it back in the oven for around 10 minutes. Then serve

Cilantro Turkey Burgers

Ingredients:

- 1 large egg, beaten well

- 2 tablespoons fresh chopped cilantro

- 1 teaspoon fresh chopped parsley

- ½ teaspoon chili powder

- 1 ½ lbs. lean ground turkey

- ¼ cup blanched almond flour

- Salt and pepper to taste

Directions:

1. Preheat your broiler to high heat.

2. Combine all of the Ingredients: in a mixing bowl and stir well.

3. Shape the mixture into six even-sized patties, pressing them to about ½-inch thick.

4. Place the patties on a broiler pan and broil for 5 minutes on each side or until cooked through.

5. Serve the burgers on lettuce wedges with your favorite burger toppings.

Bacon-Wrapped Scallops

Ingredients:

- Salt and pepper to taste

- ½ lbs. uncooked bacon, strips cut in half

- 1 lbs. large sea scallops

- ½ teaspoon chili powder

- Pinch of cayenne

Directions:

1. Preheat your broiler to high heat.
2. Rinse the scallops with cool water and pat dry with paper towel.
3. Place the scallops on a broiler pan and sprinkle with chili powder, cayenne, salt and pepper.
4. Wrap each scallop with a half slice of bacon and secure the strips in place with toothpicks.

5. Broil the scallops for 5 to 10 minutes until they are cooked through and the bacon is crisp.

Oven-Roasted Rosemary Chicken

Ingredients:

- 2 large yellow onions, sliced

- 2 tablespoons dried rosemary

- ¼ cup chicken broth

- 3 lbs. b2-in chicken legs

- 2 tablespoons olive oil

- Salt and pepper to taste

Directions:

1. Preheat the oven to 400°F.
2. Heat the oil in a large skillet over medium-high heat.
3. Season the chicken with salt and pepper to taste then add to the skillet.
4. Cook for 3 to 4 minutes on each side until browned.

5. Spread the onions in the bottom of a glass baking dish.
6. Place the chicken on top, skin-side down, and sprinkle with rosemary.
7. Drizzle the chicken with chicken broth and roast for 30 minutes.
8. Flip the chicken and roast for another 25 to 30 minutes until the juices run clear.

Coconut Flapjacks

Ingredients:

- 1 teaspoon baking soda

- 3 eggs

- ½ cup almond or container assortment coconut milk

- ½ cup water

- 1 teaspoon vanilla

- 2 tablespoons butter, dissolved

- ¼ cup coconut flour

- ¼ cup almond meal

- 1 tablespoon xylitol or ¼ teaspoon fluid stevia or to wanted sweetness discretionary

Directions:

1. Preheat a frying pan over medium warmth. In an expansive dish, consolidate the coconut flour, almond dinner, and baking soda. In a little bowl, whisk the eggs.
2. Include the milk, water, vanilla, butter, and xylitol or stevia on the off chance that utilizing, and whisk well.
3. Empty the egg mixture into the flour mixture and blend until consolidated.
4. Oil a skillet or frying pan and warm over medium warmth.
5. For every pancake, pour ¼ cup of batter onto the frying pan.
6. Cook for 2 to 3 minutes, or until the air pockets structure and the edges are cooked.
7. Turn and cook for 2 minutes, or until the underside are daintily seared. Rehash with the remaining batter.

Chopped Chicken Hash

Ingredients:

- ¼ cup onion, cleaved

- 1 medium tomato, hacked

- ½ cup red bell pepper, seeded and slashed

- ½ cup cooked grass-nourished chicken, hacked

- 1 ½ teaspoons additional virgin coconut oil

- 2 cloves garlic, slashed

- 2-3 turnips, peeled and hacked into 3D squares

- ½ cup spinach, trimmed and torn

Directions:

1. Flaked ocean salt and black pepper, to taste

2. In a non-stick pan, warm oil on medium warmth. Include onion and sauté for around 1 moment.

3. Include turnip and cook blending regularly for around 5 minutes. Include onion, tomato and bell pepper and cook, mixing regularly for 5 minutes. Include chicken and cook for 4 to 5 minutes.

4. Include spinach and cook for 2 to 3 minutes or until simply shriveled.

5. Season with salt and black pepper. Serve this hash with poached eggs.

Pancakes With Lemon-Poppy Seeds

Ingredients:

- 1 tablespoon naturally ground lemon peel

- 2 teaspoons poppy seeds

- ¼ teaspoon lemon stevia or to fancied sweetness discretionary

- 1½ cups whitened almond flour

- ½ teaspoon baking powder

- ¼ teaspoon baking soda

- 3 vast eggs, isolated

- 4 tablespoons buttermilk

- 1 tablespoon lemon juice

- ¼ teaspoon ocean salt

Directions:

1. In a vast dish, whisk together the egg yolks, buttermilk, lemon juice, lemon peel, poppy seeds, and stevia if utilizing.

2. Include the almond flour, baking powder, baking soda, and salt and mix until completely joined.

3. In a little bowl, whisk the egg whites until marginally hardened.

4. Fold into the batter. Oil a skillet or frying pan and warm over medium warmth.

5. For every pancake, scoop 2 piling tablespoons of batter onto the skillet.

6. Cook for 1-2 minutes, or until air pockets structure around the edges.

7. Turn and cook for 1 minute, or until underside is delicately cooked.

8. Uproot to a serving platter.

9. Rehash with the remaining batter, re-lubing the skillet if required.

Bay Infused Shallots

Ingredients:

- 3 tablespoons of olive oil

- 2 tablespoons of balsamic vinegar

- 500g shallots

- 4 bay leaves

- A dozen black olives

Directions:

1. Heat the oven to 350F. Submerge the shallots in boiling water and leave for a moment.

2. Next, remove the shallots and peel them. If any shallot is particularly large, cut it in half.

3. Place the shallots in an ovenproof dish.

4. Add the bay leaves and balsamic vinegar and then drizzle with the 3 tablespoons of olive oil and a pinch of salt.

5. Bake for 35 minutes, stirring the mixture and adding the olives halfway through.

Mediterranean Couscous

Ingredients:

- 140g pitted black olives

- 140g sundried tomatoes

- Fresh parsley

- 12 cherry tomatoes

- Dash of lemon juice

- 400g couscous

- 2 tablespoons of olive oil

- 500g soft dried apricots

- 1 zucchini

- 1 yellow bell pepper

Directions:

1. Chop and de-seed all the fruit and vegetables.

2. Pour the couscous into a mixing bowl and add 700ml of boiling water.

3. Cover the mixing bowl and leave for 10 minutes.

4. Add the olive oil and parsley, with a dash of lemon juice.

5. Using a fork, break and fluff the couscous.

6. Combine the fruit and vegetables into the mixing bowl and serve.

Pecan Caramel Cookie Bark

Ingredients:

For The Caramel Sauce:

- 1 cup full fat coconut milk

- 1 cup maple sugar

- 1 teaspoon vanilla extract

- 1/4 teaspoon salt

For The Bark:

- 1/3 cup toasted pecans

- 1 cup mini chocolate chips, melted + extra for garnishing

- 7-8 gluten free pecan cookies

Directions:

Make Caramel Sauce:

1. Combine all the Ingredients: in a small saucepan.
2. Place the saucepan over medium heat and stir until completely combined.
3. Once combined, bring to a boil for 12 minutes, ensuring the mixture doesn't boil over.
4. After 12 minutes, lower the heat to a simmer for an additional 5 minutes, or until the caramel lightly coats the back of a spoon.
5. Remove from the heat and let the mixture cool for 5 minutes.
6. Preheat the oven to 350F. Place the pecans on a baking sheet and roast in over for 10 minutes or until dark and fragrant.
7. Keep an eye on them so they don't burn.
8. As the pecans are roasting, melt the chocolate in a double boiler or in the microwave.

9. Be careful not to burn. Once the chocolate is melted, pour the chocolate on a parchment paper lined baking sheet and spread evenly.

10. Add the cookies and toasted pecans to the melted chocolate.

11. The next step is to use a spoon to spread the caramel throughout the chocolate.

12.

13. Finally, sprinkle the chocolate chips on top. Place the prepared chocolate in the freezer for about 30 minutes to harden. Remove from freezer and break into pieces.

Cookie Dough Bites

Ingredients:

- ¾ cup cassava flour

- pinch of salt

- ½ cup mini chocolate chips

- 2 cups mini chocolate chips or whatever chocolate you prefer, melted

- ½ cup softened coconut oil

- ½ cup maple sugar

- 1 teaspoon vanilla extract

Directions:

1. Cream together the coconut oil, sugar and vanilla extract with a hand mixer.

2. Slowly add the cassava flour while the mixer is running until all the flour is combined.
3. Fold in the salt and chocolate chips. Using a spoon or cookie scoop, shape the dough into 12-14 balls.
4. Place the balls in the fridge for 10-15 minutes in order to harden.
5. Melt the chocolate in a microwave or double boiler, being careful not to burn.
6. Using a fork, dip each cookie dough ball into the chocolate and coat all sides.
7. Places the balls in the fridge to harden for about 10 minutes.
8. Bring the balls to room temperature before serving. Serve with a toothpick.

Strawberry Dark Chocolate Chunk Cookies

Ingredients:

- 1 tablespoons coconut flour

- 1 teaspoon baking soda

- 1 teaspoon vanilla extract

- pinch of salt

- 3 ounce chocolate bar, roughly chopped

- 1 cup raw almond butter

- 1 cup maple sugar

- 1 egg

- 1 tablespoon tapioca flour

- 1/3 cup dried strawberries

Directions:

1. Preheat oven to 350F and line a baking sheet with parchment paper.

2. In a large mixing bowl, stir together the almond butter and maple sugar.

3. Then add beaten egg. After mixture is combined, add the tapioca and coconut flour, baking soda, vanilla, salt and chocolate chunks. Mix to thoroughly combine.

4. Using a cookie scoop or spoon, create about 2 tablespoons of dough into a ball. Place on baking sheet. Press a dried strawberry or 3 into each cookie.

5. Place baking sheet in oven and bake for 10 minutes.

6. Remove from oven and let cool for 10 minutes.

7. If you try to transfer to cooling rack too soon, they will come apart.

Pineapple Tapioca

Ingredients:

- Tapioca, 1 cup.

- Pineapple juice, 1 cup.

- Water, 4 cups.

- Sugar, 2-3 cup.

Directions:

1. Better results take after when the tapioca is splashed over night or for a few hours.

2. Wash the tapioca, and splash in the water; just before cooking include sugar and pineapple juice.

3. Cook in a 3fold boiler until straightforward, and pour into a level dish to cool.

4. On the off chance that cut pineapple is within reach, dice it, and place in the base of the dish, before pouring in the tapioca.

5. On the off chance that, when cooking tapioca or sago for pudding, it ought to cook too long and get flimsy, it might be made into a decent pastry by beating it into beaten egg whites; season, and shape in cups or dish. Present with a hued sauce.

Cheese Fondue

Ingredients:

- 1 clove garlic, divided

- 1 cup chicken puree

- 3 ounces cream cheese, cut into lumps

- 2 cups destroyed Gruyère cheese 8 ounces

- 2 cups destroyed Swiss cheese 8 ounces

- 1 tablespoon arrowroot

- ½ teaspoon dry mustard

Directions:

1. In a medium dish, hurl the Gruyere and Swiss with the arrowroot and mustard until covered.
2. Rub the garlic parts all around within the highest point of a 3fold boiler, and then toss.
3. Add the chicken puree to the 3fold boiler and place over stewing water.
4. Step by step include the cheese mixture, blending until the cheeses are dissolved.
5. Mix in the cream cheese just until softened.
6. Expel from the warmth. Keep warm in a fondue pot while serving.

Petite Raisin-White Chocolate

Ingredients:

- ½ cup of margarine, softened

- ¾ cup raisins, cleaved coarsely

- ¾ cup whipping cream

- 2 teaspoons of shortening

- 1 ¼ cups of white baking chocolate chips ideally gluten-free

- 2 cups sans wheat flour mix

- 1/3 cup of sugar

- 1 teaspoon of lemon zing, newly ground

- 2 teaspoons of baking powder

- ½ teaspoon of salt

Directions:

1. For the flour mix, join 2/3 cups of potato starch, 1 teaspoon of thickener, 2 cups of rice flour, and 1/3 cup of custard flour. Utilize just the required measure of flour mix for this formula. Mix everything again before using.

2. Preheat the stove to 400 degrees Fahrenheit.

3. Combine the baking powder, salt, flour mix, sugar, and lemon zing in a huge bowl. Include the margarine utilizing a baked good blender or a fork.

4. The resulting combination will take after coarse crumbs.

5. Add in the whipping cream. Blend everything great until the batter is strong.

6. Include the raisins and ¾ cup of the white baking chocolate chips.

7. On a daintily floured surface, turn the batter.

8. Work it for around 5-10 times or until the batter is smooth.

9. Partition it into 4 equivalent parts.

10. Make each or until the batter is smooth.
    Partition it into 4 equivalent parts.

11. Make each inch pieces 4 sections, and
    afterward cut every 2 of the squares slantingly
    in half to make little triangles.

12. On an ungreased baking sheet, place the sc2s
    no less than an inch separated.

13. Heat the sc2s for around 9-11 minutes until
    the edges become brilliant brown. Cool them
    completely.

14. Combine the shortening and the leftover
    baking chips in a microwaveable bowl.

15. Microwave the blend on medium, for around
    30 seconds.

16. Mix and keep on microwaving until the blend
    becomes smooth and totally softened.

17. Sprinkle the highest point of the sc2s with the
    liquefied chocolate.

Patatas Braves Spicy Potatoes

Ingredients:

- 4-5 garlic cloves

- 1 8-ounce container of tomato sauce

- 1 ½ teaspoons of sherry vinegar

- Heaping ¼ teaspoon squashed red pepper

- ½ teaspoon paprika

- 1 pound reddish brown potatoes, or

- 3 medium potatoes

- ¼ teaspoon ocean salt

- 4 teaspoons olive oil, divided

Directions:

1. Cut potatoes in half the long way, then, at that point, cut every half again longwise.

2. Cut into fragments that are ½ inch in size.

3. Over medium hotness, heat a huge skillet. Add around 2 teaspoons of olive oil.

4. When the oil is hot, add the salt and the potatoes.

5. Mix well, and afterward spread the potatoes well in a solitary layer.

6. Every 5-10 minutes, give the potatoes a mix and scratch the dish.

7. Assuming you see that the potatoes are turning out to be too brown outwardly, you can bring down the hotness medium-low.

8. Cook until the potatoes become firm and brown outwardly and delicate inside.

9. It requires around 45 minutes to an hour.

10. While the potatoes are cooking, mince the garlic finely.

11. On medium hotness, heat a little pan and add 2 teaspoons of olive oil.
12. Once hot, add the garlic in the little pot and sauté for about a moment.

    -Then, at that point, add the vinegar, pureed tomatoes, and flavors.
13. Mix well and afterward bring down the hotness.
14. Stew for around 20 minutes to 30 minutes in low hotness. Once d2, eliminate the dish from the heat.
15. Once the potatoes are cooked, top them with the sauce and serve right away.

Cabbage Roll Casserole

Ingredients:

- 1 3/4 pounds chopped cabbage

- 1/2 cup uncooked white rice

- 1/2 teaspoon salt

- 1 14 oz. can beef broth

- 1 pound ground beef

- 1/2 cup chopped onion

- 1 28 oz. can tomato sauce

Directions:

1. Preheat oven to 350 degrees F.

2. In a large skillet, brown the beef in oil over medium heat until the redness disappears. Drain fat.

3. In a large bowl, mix the onion, tomatoes, cabbage, rice and salt.

4. Add meat and mix well. Pour mixture in a 9x13 inch baking pan.

5. Pour the broth over the covered meat mixture and bake in preheated oven for 1 hour.

6. Stir, put the lid back and cook for 30 minutes.

Mushroom Risotto

Ingredients:

- 1 ½ cups sliced fresh mushrooms

- 1 cup whole milk

- ¼ cup heavy cream

- 1 cup rice

- 5 cups vegetable stock

- 1 teaspoon butter

- 1 tablespoon olive oil

- 3 small onions, chopped

- 1 clove garlic, minced

- 1 teaspoon fresh parsley

- 1 teaspoon minced celery

- salt and pepper to taste

- 1 cup grated Parmesan cheese

Directions:

1. Take a pan, add olive oil on medium-high heat.
2. Deep fry onion and garlic until the onion is soft and garlic lightly browned.
3. Remove the garlic and stir in parsley, celery, salt and pepper.
4. Cook until celery is tender, then the mushrooms. Reduce heat and continue cooking until the mushrooms are soft.
5. Pour the milk and cream into the pan and whirl in the rice.
6. Simmer and stir the vegetable stock into the rice 2 cup at a time, until it is absorbed.
7. When the rice is finished cooking, mix the butter and Parmesan, and remove from heat. Serve warm.

Meringue Pops

Ingredients:

- 1 tsp.vanilla extract

- 1 cup sweetener

- 4 egg whites

- A pinch of cream of tartar

Directions:

1. Preheat oven at 175°F.
2. Whisk the egg whites, sweetener, and tartar in a bowl over simmering water.
3. Pour the mixture into another bowl and then continue blending using an electronic hand held mixture on slow speed.
4. Add the vanilla extract and then increase the speed.
5. Continue mixing until the mixture stiffens and creates peaks.

6. Transfer mixture in a pastry bag and then pipe the egg white mixture on a baking sheet lined with parchment paper.
7. Bake for 1½hours and let it cool before serving.
8. You can store the meringue in airtight containers away from heat or moisture.

Wheat-Free Carrot Cupcakes

Ingredients:

- 2 tsp. cinnamon ground

- 1 cup pecans chopped

- ½tsp. grated nutmeg

- ½tsp sea salt

- 2 tsbp. orange peel

- 2 eggs separate yolks and whites

- ½cup sour cream

- 1 cup carrots shredded

- 1½cups almond flour

- 1½tsp. baking powder

- 1 tsp. baking soda

- ¼tsp. cream of tartar

- ½cup flaxseed ground

- ¼cup organic butter melted

- ½cup applesauce

Directions:

1. Preheat oven at 350˚F.

2. Place the almond flour, chopped pecans, cinnamon, baking powder, baking soda, flax seeds, stevia, nutmeg, and salt in a mixing bowl and combine.

3. Add the carrots and orange peel and mix.

4. In a separate bowl, whisk the yolks, sour cream, melted butter, and apple sauce.

5. In another bowl, whish the egg whites and cream of tartar using an electronic mixer until it becomes stiff or when peaks form.

6. Gently add in the mixture with yolks and fold gently.

7. Add the egg mixture into the dry Ingredients:
    and fold gently.
8. Scoop the batter into 12-16 cups and bake for
    about 40 mins. Let it cool for 5 mins. and
    serve.

Balsamic Chicken And Bacon Wraps

Ingredients:

- 4 ounces of Portobello mushrooms sliced

- 2 tablespoons of balsamic vinegar

- 4 flaxseed wraps recipe can be found above

- 2 tablespoons of EVOO extra virgin olive oil

- 1 piece of chicken breast skinless and b2less; cut to strips

- 4 slices of bacon thick-cut

- 2 cups of romaine lettuce shredded

Directions:

1. Using a large pan, heat oil over medium to high heat. Cook the chicken, mushrooms and bacon for about 8 minutes or until chicken is thoroughly cooked.
2. Make sure that the bacon is also cooked and mushrooms are already golden brown.
3. Using a slotted spoon, transfer bacon and chicken into a plate leaving mushroom on the pan. Set aside the bacon and chicken.
4. Reduce heat and add vinegar on the mushroom.
5. Simmer and stir for about a minute or until vinegar is reduced. Take it out of the stove.
6. Lay wraps in a plate. Arrange bacon and chicken and top with mushroom mixture and wraps. Roll it up.
7. Serve and enjoy!

Roasted Cauliflower With Spiced Almonds

Ingredients:

- 2 teaspoons of cumin

- 2 teaspoons of coriander seeds

- 1-2 pieces of dried chillies

- A handful of almonds blanched and smashed

- 1 head of cauliflower leaves removed and broken down to florets

- 1 knob of butter

- 1 lemon juiced and zest needed

Directions:

1. Preheat oven to 400 degrees F.

2. Blanch cauliflower in boiling water with salt. Drain and dry.

3. Don't allow any water to be left. This will not allow the cauliflower to roast well.

4. Transfer to a bowl and add butter and olive oil. Toss to coat evenly.

5. Using your pestle and mortar, pound chillies and spices and add a bit of salt.

6. Mix them with almonds and place on a dry and hot ovenproof tray or pan and slowly toast them.

7. Add cauliflower. Once cauliflower has color, add lemon juice and zest.

8. Mix well to coat evenly. Fry for 1 minute then place it inside the oven and cook around 15 minutes until crisp.

9. Serve and enjoy!

Classic Pizza

Ingredients:

- 4 tablespoons of golden flaxseed ground

- 1 teaspoon of powdered onion

- ½ teaspoon of powdered garlic

- ½ teaspoon of sea salt

- 2 large sized eggs

- 1 cup of mozzarella cheese Shredded

- 2 cups of walnut or pecan meal

- ¼ cup of garbanzo beans you can also use coconut flour

- 4 tablespoons of EVOO extra virgin olive oil

- ½ cup of water

Directions:

1. Preheat your oven to 350 degrees F.

2. Using a food chopper or processor, chop/pulse the mozzarella cheese until it becomes granular in size.

3. Using a large bowl, mix almond flour, ground flaxseed, powdered onion, garbanzo bean, powdered garlic and salt. Add mozzarella cheese, eggs, water and olive oil. Combine well.

4. Line a large cookie sheet using a parchment paper. Place the mixture on the parchment paper and coat your hands with olive oil. Knead the mixture until it forms a dough. Form according to your desired shape.

5. Using another parchment paper, spread it on top of the dough and use a rolling pin to flatten. Form according to preferred shape and feel if desired thickness is okay. Remove

the parchment paper and discard. Bake for about 20 minutes. Remove from oven.

6. Top the crust with your favorite toppings. Add tomato sauce then mozzarella cheese and other veggies and meat available. Drizzle with olive oil.

7. Bake for another 15 minutes or until you can see that the cheese is already melted and crust is golden brown.

8. Slice, serve and enjoy!

Zucchini "Pasta"

Ingredients:

- Tomato sauce 1 cup

- extra-virgin olive oil 4 tablespoons

- Parmesan cheese 1/4 cup, grated

- Garlic cloves 3 pieces, minced

- Fresh basil 2 tablespoons, chopped

- Salt a pinch

- Zucchini 1 pound

- Meat of your choice; Sausage, turkey, ground beef, chicken, or pork 8 ounces

- Black pepper a pinch, ground

Directions:

1. Using a vegetable peeler, peel the zucchini.
2. Then, cut the zucchini lengthwise to form ribbons until you get to the seed core.
3. Get a large skillet and grease it with 1 tablespoon of oil. Add the ribb2d zucchini and cook for 4-5 minutes.
4. In a separate pan, cook the meat for 5 minutes. Make sure to drain off the fat.
5. Add the garlic and cook for another 2-3 minutes.
6. Lay the ribb2d zucchini on the plate and place the meat on top and serve.

Pot Roast

Ingredients:

- 1 tsp. Of black pepper, freshly ground

- 2 tbsp. Of extra virgin olive oil

- 2 lb. Of grass-fed beef chuck steak

- 1 cup of beef stock or red wine

- 4 cloves of garlic, coarsely chopped

- 2 large onions, sliced thinly

- 1 tsp. Of dry thyme

- 1 tbsp. Of paprika

- 1 tsp. Of dry rosemary

- Sea salt

Directions:-

1. Combine the herbs and spices together in a bowl to make the spice rub.
2. Generously rub it into the beef.
3. For the best flavor time permitting, you can leave the meat in the refrigerator overnight.
4. 3 Preheat oven at 350 degrees.
5. In a heavy casserole or Dutch oven, heat olive oil on medium-high heat.
6. Sear the meat till brown on all sides; this will take about a minute per side.
7. Remove the roast temporarily by putting it on a plate.
8. Remove the excess fat in the pan. Add stock, water, or wine to pan; de-glaze by scraping down and dissolving brown bits on bottom.
9. Return the beef to Dutch oven, cover with garlic and sliced onions, cover and bake it in the oven for an hour.

10. Turn the roast over and continue cooking for another hour, uncovered.

11. Add extra liquid if necessary; stir onions after 30 minutes for an even cooking.

12. Cover the pan again; cook for 1 more hour. The beef will be cooked once it is fork tender.

13. Remove meat from pot; allow it to rest covered loosely with foil.

14. Season the sauce with pepper and salt if desired. Serve sauce over meat after plating.

Almond Parmesan Haddock

Ingredients:

- 2 tablespoons finely chopped almonds

- Salt and pepper to taste

- 1 large egg, beaten well

- 4 6-ounce b2less haddock fillets

- ¼ cup blanched almond flour

- ¼ cup grated parmesan cheese

Directions:

1. Preheat the oven to 350°F and line a baking sheet with parchment.
2. Combine the almond flour, almonds and parmesan cheese in a shallow dish.
3. Beat the egg in another dish and set it aside.

4. Season the fillets with salt and pepper to taste then dip them in the egg.
5. Dredge the fillets in the almond parmesan mixture then place them on the baking sheet.
6. Bake for 12 to 15 minutes until the flesh flakes easily with a fork.
7. Serve the fillets hot with lemon wedges.

Herbed Pork Tenderloin

Ingredients:

- 1 tablespoon fresh chopped rosemary

- 2 teaspoons fresh chopped thyme

- ½ teaspoon fresh chopped oregano

- 2 1-lbs. b2less pork tenderloins

- ½ cup fresh lemon juice

- 1 tablespoon minced garlic

- Salt and pepper to taste

Directions:

1. Combine all of the Ingredients: except for the tenderloin in a mixing bowl and stir until well combined.

2. Place the tenderloins in a zippered freezer bag and pour in the marinade.
3. Shake to coat then chill for at least 3 hours
4. Preheat the oven to 400°F and line a roasting pan with foil.
5. Season the tenderloins with salt and pepper to taste and place them on the roasting pan.
6. Roast the tenderloins for 12 to 15 minutes or until the internal temperature reaches 140°F.
7. Cover the tenderloins in foil and let rest for 10 minutes before slicing.

Coconut-Almond Crunchy Pancakes

Ingredients:

- ½ cup almond milk

- ¼ cup almond butter, liquefied

- 4 unfenced eggs, beaten

- 1 teaspoon crisp lemon squeeze

- 1 tablespoon normal stevia

- ½ cup coconut flour

- ½ cup almond flour

- ½ teaspoon non-aluminium baking soda

- ¼ cup almonds, hacked Extra-virgin coconut oil, for cooking

Directions:

1. In a dish, include flours and baking soda and mix well. In another dish, include butter and milk and beat well.

2. Include eggs, lemon squeeze and Stevia and beat until very much consolidated.

3. Mix egg mixture into flour mixture.

4. Crease in cleaved almonds. In a huge skillet, warm oil on medium warmth. Include a mixture in sought size.

5. Cook for 3 to 4 minutes for each side.

6. Rehash with the remaining mixture. Present with almond or peanut butter.

Grilled Cheese Bake

Ingredients:

- 2 cups inexactly pressed infant spinach

- 2 tomatoes, cut into 8 cuts

- 4 eggs

- 1½ cups creamer

- ½ teaspoon nutmeg

- 1 teaspoon ocean salt

- 14 cuts ½" thick wheat free Basic Bread from the first section

- 2 cups destroyed Fontina or Gruyère cheese, partiti2d

- ½ teaspoon ground black pepper

Directions:

1. Preheat the oven to 375°F. Oil a 9" × 9" baking pan with butter.
2. Toast the bread in a toaster on medium setting.
3. Line the base of the baking pan with 7 cuts, slicing to fit.
4. Sprinkle with 1 cup of the cheese, then top with the spinach. Top with the tomatoes.
5. Pivot the pan 45 degrees and spot the remaining 7 cuts of bread transversely to the first so that the bread is not stacked like a sandwich.
6. Sprinkle the remaining 1 cup cheese over the bread.
7. In a medium dish, whisk the eggs and cream until the yolks are separated. Include the nutmeg, salt, and pepper, and rush to join.
8. Pour over the bread, making a point to splash every last bit of it.

9. Spread with foil and prepare for 20 minutes.

10. Evacuate the foil and prepare for 25 minutes, or until the eggs are puffy and the cheese is sautéed.

11. In the event that the cheese tans before the eggs set, swap the foil for the last minutes. Let stand for 10 minutes prior to serving.

Thyme & Mustard Roasted New Potatoes

Ingredients:

- 3 tablespoons of extra-virgin olive oil

- 1 tablespoon of wholegrain mustard

- 1.25 kg of new potatoes

- 3 thyme sprigs

Directions:

1. Preheat the oven to 450F or gas mark 8. Halve the new potatoes.

2. Evenly place the new potatoes on a baking tray.

3. Garnish with 2 tablespoons of olive oil, thyme sprigs and a pinch of salt. Bake for 50 minutes.

4. Serve with a drizzle of 1 tablespoon of olive oil and mustard. This is an excellent dish to accompany a salad.

Squash & Fig Curry

Ingredients:

- 100g red lentils

- 2 teaspoons of brown sugar

- 2 teaspoons of white wine vinegar

- 400g kidney beans

- 2 dried figs

- ½ bunch parsley

- 400g butternut squash

- 1 onion

- 1 tablespoon of olive oil

- 2 teaspoons of cumin

- ½ teaspoon of chilli flakes

- 400g chopped tomatoes

- 150ml of soy yogurt

Directions:

1. Peel and dice the squash. Peel and slice the onion.
2. Dice the figs into small pieces and chop the parsley.
3. In a large skillet, briefly heat 1 tablespoon of olive oil.
4. Add the squash and onion, and then fry until the onion has become golden and soft.
5. Add in the cumin and chilli, then stir and fry for another 2 minutes.
6. Next, combine the lentils, brown sugar and white wine vinegar to the skillet mixture, alongside a cup of water, then fry for another 2 minutes.
7. Leave to simmer for a final 10 minutes, before adding in the kidney beans and heating them for a brief moment.

8. Combine the figs with the soy yogurt and parsley. Serve the fig mixture with the curry.

Chocolate Truffles

Ingredients:

- 1 cup full-fat coconut milk

- 1 teaspoon vanilla extract

- ½ cup finely shredded unsweetened coconut and/or ½ cup unsweetened cocoa

- 10 ounces dark chocolate, 70% cacao content or higher

- 3 tablespoons coconut oil

Directions:
1. Place the shredded chocolate and coconut oil in a medium bowl.
2. Set aside for later. In a small saucepan over medium heat, heat the coconut milk until simmering.

3. Once the milk has reached its temperature, pour over the chocolate and coconut mixture.

4. Stir gently with a spatula or spoon to combine.

5. Don't mix too quickly in order to protect the chocolate from becoming grainy.

6. Add the vanilla and stir to combine.

7. Transfer the mixture to a sealed container and chill until solid at least 4 hours.

8. Lightly toast the shredded coconut on a parchment-lined baking tray at 300°F oven for 3 to 5 minutes or until golden brown.

9. Move the flakes to a bowl in order to allow them to cool.

10. Once the chocolate mixture has chilled in the fridge, scoop out 36 balls of chocolate.

11. Roll each ball between your palms to form a smooth ball.

12. Coat the truffle with the toasted coconut. Alternatively, you can use sifted cocoa powder.

No-Bake Pumpkin Bars

Ingredients:

- 5 oz. unsweetened coconut flakes, plus more for garnish

- 1 tablespoon coconut oil, melted

- 1/2 teaspoon vanilla extract

- Pinch of salt

- 1/3 cup pumpkin puree

- 10 pitted Medjool dates

- 1 cup almonds

- 1 1/2 tablespoons dark unsweetened cocoa powder

- 2 teaspoons cinnamon, divided

- 1/2 banana

- 2 tablespoon h2y

Directions:

1. Cover dates with water in a bowl.

2. Allow to soak for 20-30 minutes to allow for softening. In the meantime, line a 9x5-inch loaf pan with wax paper. In a food processor, place the almonds and pulse to finely chop.

3. Add the soaked dates drain soaking water, cocoa powder, and 1 teaspoon of cinnamon.

4. Blend the Ingredients: and the processor until rough dough starts to form.

5. Transfer the dough to the loaf pan and flatten evenly with a spatula.

6. Place the coconut flakes, coconut oil, salt and vanilla in the food processor and mix for at least 1 minute until a paste starts to form.

7. Add this mixture to the loaf pan, spreading evenly over the almond mixture base.

8. Add to the food processor, the pumpkin puree, banana, h2y and remaining teaspoon of cinnamon. Blend until smooth.

9. Spread this mixture evenly over the coconut mixture in the loaf pan.

10. Sprinkle with coconut flakes if preferred.

11. Place in freezer for 1 hour. Cut into squares before serving.

Teriyaki Eggplant Steaks

Ingredients:

- ¼ cup mirin or dry white wine or sake

- ¼ cup water

- 1/3 cup tamari or soy sauce gluten-free

- 1 garlic clove enormous, minced

- 2 little scallions or green onions, minced

- 3 little eggplants globe, with the stems taken out and the eggplants cut transversely to about ½ inch thick

- a piece of ginger around 1 ½ inches long, minced

- Crushed red pepper a pinch

Directions:

1. Combine everything in a pan, aside from the eggplants.
2. At the point when it approaches medium hotness, pass on the blend to stew for around 10 minutes. The sauce will become thicker.
3. Once d2, eliminate from the heat.
4. Put the eggplant cuts inside a meal dish. Cover it with the sauce. Leave the eggplants in the marinade for around 1-2 hours, turning them occasionally.
5. Using a frying pan dish or an enormous skillet, heat over medium-high hotness.
6. Put oil until the dish is recorded softly. Lay the eggplants on the dish and fry until seared softly.
7. Flip and afterward cook for a couple of more minutes.

8. Remove eggplants from hotness and put away.

9. Do similar interaction with the excess eggplants all have been completely cooked. Serve.